Juice With Me

A Beginner's Guide

By TL Bliss

Table of Contents

Introduction

At this moment, today, how do you feel about your life, your weight, what you eat daily, and more importantly your overall wellbeing? Have you ever been inspired to change your life around to take all of these needs and make them work for you? Have you tried to lose weight and it just did not work? Have you tried to eat better meals and it also did not work? I was in the same situation and answered yes to these questions, just like you. I want to assure you - there is hope and I documented this hope to share with you here. The answer comes in the form of juice.

Earlier this year, I realized that I needed to start paying closer attention to my health, diet, and especially my weight. I wanted to change my life around and make all of my needs work for me. I watched a documentary by Joe Cross, which is titled, "*Fat, Sick, and Nearly Dead*", and little did I know it would change my life. After watching this documentary, I told my husband that I was going to research the information I learned and gain better knowledge of how and why the concept of juicing worked. Was there a cure for junk food syndrome after all?

When I began my juice fast, I documented my beginning measurements as:

> *Bust line: 42 inches*
> *Belly button waistline: 44 inches*
> *Hips: 47 inches*
> *Left leg girth: 27 inches*
> *Right leg girth: 28 inches*
> *Weight: 194 pounds.*

Another set of measurements after beginning my juicing journey:

> *Bust line: 41 inches*
> *Belly button waistline: 43 inches*
> *Hips: 47 inches*
> *Left leg girth: 27 inches*
> *Right leg girth: 28 inches*
> *Weight: 190 pounds.*

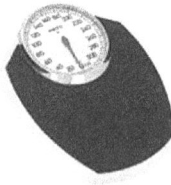

Still going strong on the juice:

> *Bust line: 38.5 inches*
> *Belly button waistline: 42 inches*
> *Hips: 46 inches*
> *Left leg girth: 27 inches*
> *Right leg girth: 27 inches*
> *Weight: 182 pounds.*

One last set of measurements I took in March while juicing:

> *Bust line: 38 inches*
> *Belly button waistline: 39 inches*
> *Hips: 44 inches*
> *Left leg girth: 26 inches*
> *Right leg girth: 27 inches*
> *Weight: 178 pounds.*

Did you notice the downward trend in all of my measurements? In only a few short months, my body was changing, slimming, getting healthier, cleansing from the inside out, and getting rid of 40 plus years of damage that I had done to it. I also did not do a continuous juice fast for three months; I started with a three-day fast, then went to a one-week fast, then added one meal a day into my juicing regimen. I bounced between juicing for three days and seven days at a time. I was able to keep my weight off and maintain my healthy new lifestyle with little to no effort. I also managed to keep those numbers down after spending 10 days on vacation at the beach. I learned that eating fruits and vegetables the right way could lead to results that are more beneficial and junk food was no longer a part of my life. I was truly inspired to eat healthier and stay away from eating junk food.

Granted my age plays a role, as do health-related issues of an aging female in maintaining my "girlish" figure. I also realize now that was only an excuse my mind tried to get *me* to believe. I was no longer willing to accept the fact that I could not do anything to change my eating habits and feel better during the process. I was not going to allow myself to continue on the nutritional path I had been on for so many years.

My diet before watching *"Fat, Sick, and Nearly Dead"* consisted of not eating breakfast, grabbing a quick burger from the more famous fast food chains, and my dinner consisted of fried foods mostly. I drank milk and ate dairy products almost daily. I also ate large portions of meat, which I no longer do.

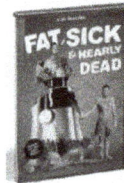

Little did I know that what I was eating, prior to watching *"Fat, Sick, and Nearly Dead"*, was literally killing me.

I grew up with the concept that drinking milk was good for me and healthy too, but sure enough, it was not. Along with drinking milk, eating meat was supposed to make me stronger, but in fact was almost worse than drinking milk. I spent my life eating and doing things I needed to change. How do you reverse 40 plus years of damage to your body? By drinking juice. Sounds simple enough, right? To some it is rather simple and to others not so much. I am sharing my juicing journey with you from beginning to end in hopes that it will inspire you.

Beginning Your Juice Fast

Congratulations on your decision to begin a juice fast. I realize that you are only in the thought process stage right now, but you will be juicing in no time.

To begin your juice fast, you have to understand your reason, or reasons, for wanting to start this phase of your life. These reasons can range from personal, weight loss, or even spiritual. My original reason was to give my body a break from the 40 plus years of "damage" that I had done to it. My body needed to be set free from the junk food I was abusing it with for so many years. Your reason will be your own personal aspiration of why you want or need to experience the benefits of a juice fast.

Juice fast. What does this mean? The juice in the sense of juicing is defined as the liquid contained in a fruit or vegetable. Fast means abstaining from food for a period of time.

If you combine the terms together, you are consuming the juice of fruits and vegetables, while you are abstaining from all other sorts of foods. Technically speaking, a true fast would mean that you are abstaining from all forms of food and beverage for a certain period of time.

Do not confuse this with starving yourself – you will be getting nutrients from the fruit and vegetable juice, so you are not starving your body of consuming healthy and nutritional sustenance. You are literally changing how you eat and what you eat, but either way you are still ingesting nutrients.

Another term that would be better used in this sense is cleansing. Cleansing means to make something clean or free from anything that is not clean. In essence, you are cleaning your body from the unclean ingestion you have endured for so many years. Scrubbing your cells to make them squeaky clean for a healthier you!

I will share my juicing experience with you as hassle free as possible. My goal is to point you in the right direction, answer your questions, and let you take it from there.

I, like you when I started, had tons of questions about juicing and had to educate myself to find the answers I was looking for. The internet helped me tremendously with this. There are social networking websites that offer the opinions and journeys of others who have started a juice fast. There are also varieties of websites that offer recipes for you to browse through and undoubtedly, there will be one or more that will sound amazingly good and you will want to try it. One of the best websites to go to is www.jointhereboot.com. This website has recipes and support ranging from A to Z. I kept a small notebook of the different recipes that I liked and I will share those with you in a later section here. The best way to get the answers to your questions is to educate yourself and research until you find what you are looking for. I did just that in hopes that it may save you some time. Educating yourself helps you learn the process, where to find answers, where to go for help, who to go to, and how to find what you are looking for. Being able to research is important and knowing what to look for is just as important. I have included a section dedicated to educating yourself later on in this guide.

Acquire Medical Approval

Before beginning any diet, fasting, or weight loss program, even in the most natural concept, please get medical approval from your physician. You may have health-related issues that will need to be monitored by your physician during your juice fast. While not all physicians will be very accepting of your decision to take part in a juice fast, some will encourage you to begin and gladly follow you along your course. Not everyone will be open-minded enough to accept other forms of medical treatment such as juicing and will even try to convince you that it is not a good thing to do because of your ailments, but in fact, it may be just the thing you and your body need. Please do your homework and research all of your intentions prior to making the final decision to commit to a juice fast. If you are truly convinced that a juice fast will help with your medical ailments, show your physician the information you gathered and remember to make a list of questions to take with you to your appointment. When all else fails, consult your physician for medical guidance. Do not attempt a juice fast if your ailments outweigh your advantage.

How Juicing Works

Juicing is another form of cleansing, but in a healthier sense. When you are drinking juice only and not eating greasy burgers and fries, your body is getting the time it needs away from the harmful fats and preservatives. It is able to take a break and recuperate from its normal routine.

When the fruits and vegetables have the juice removed, the juice is concentrated with micronutrients. These micronutrients are the *"cleaners"* of your body. The cleansing takes place when you consume the juice and it removes the unhealthy debris from your cells After a couple of days consuming juice, your body starts to get clean from the inside out and expels the debris from your body. This debris may come in the form of diarrhea, sweating (fevers), headaches, dizziness, little pustular red spots on your skin, and other forms of the symptoms you may experience while juicing. Once these harmful toxins are expelled from your body, then the cells can be cleansed by the micronutrients. This is when you start feeling the best. You will have a burst of energy, your thoughts will be clear, your dizziness will be gone, and you will be on the road to being healthier.

Through the many hours of research I did learning about juicing, I was able to compile this list of some of the micronutrients our bodies need every day and some of the fruits and vegetables for each micronutrient. This is not a complete list of micronutrients or fruits but hopefully enough to get you started in the right direction; all of this information can be found online and through several of the more recognized medical websites.

- Beta carotene - Found in green plants, carrots, sweet potatoes, squash, spinach, apricots, peppers, pumpkins, cantaloupe, tomatoes, radishes, watermelon, kale, leafy greens, lettuce, broccoli, brussel sprouts, and asparagus.
- Carotenoids - Found in sweet Potatoes, pumpkins, carrots, spinach, broccoli, apricots, and cantaloupe.

- Choline – Found in spinach, green leafy vegetables, peas, brussel sprouts, and legumes.
- Cryptoxanthin - Found in lemons, apples, cantaloupe, figs, grapefruit, kiwi, mangoes, peaches, pears, pineapples, tangerines, beets, sweet corn, pumpkins, squash, and carrots.
- Lutein - Found in green leafy vegetables, green colored vegetables like zucchini squash, asparagus, and broccoli.
- Lycopene - Found in tomatoes, apricots, grapefruit, and watermelon.
- Vitamin A – Helps with your immune functions, vision, reproduction, skin, teeth, and soft tissues.
- Vitamin B (all forms) - Helps with your body metabolism, energy, muscles, skin, hair, nails, immune and nervous systems.
- Vitamin C – Helps with make collagen which is needed to heal wounds, works as an antioxidant, supports your immune system, and helps your body absorb calcium.
- Vitamin D – Strengthen your bones by helping the body absorb calcium, and helps your immune function.
- Vitamin E – Helps your body make red blood cells, helps promote scar healing, and is an antioxidant.
- Vitamin K – Helps with blood clotting, aids with insulin sensitivity, and helps your cardiovascular system.

Buying A Juicer

To begin with, when it comes to preparing your purchases for juicing, again there is homework and research that you will need to do. Are you looking to juice, make smoothies, or blend? These are all different types of extracting and each has their own culinary advantage. Juicers have a wide range of makers and prices. They can be purchased online or at department stores. Purchasing a juicer can be easy and fun. Purchase one that will clean easily as you will be using it every day and cleaning it every day as well. With that being said, purchase a juicer durable enough to sustain the length of your juicing goal. There are multiple online websites to make your purchase or shop at one of your local stores to get the best deals in town. There are some juicers that are better than others, some will look nice and cost quite a bit of money, but it will eventually come down to what suits your needs and your finances. There is not one single juicer that is an absolute requirement; go with what fits your needs.

Buying Your Fruits And Vegetables For Juicing

Fruits and vegetables can be purchased anywhere you would normally shop for groceries. They can be purchased at local farmers markets, groceries stores, roadside produce stands, online retailers, and local produce stands as well. If you are looking to purchase something that is out of season in your local area, you can find a variety of online organic and nonorganic fruit and vegetable suppliers. Purchasing fruits and vegetables is a personal preference and there is not any one single place to buy your supplies; it all depends on where you want to shop and what is available to you.

Growing Your Own Supplies

Growing your own fruits and vegetables is actually the preferred method of acquiring your supplies, but realistically we are not all able to do so. Those who live in apartment buildings may not have any outdoor space to grow anything, while others may have tons of acreage for growing their own unlimited supply of fruits and vegetables. Growing your own organic food supplies ensures the quality of your produce and growing locally provides natural resources for you and your family.

Definition of Organic

While most of the time, we buy our fruits and vegetables from the grocery store, it is preferred to get them freshly grown from either your own garden or another produce garden. The store bought supplies will need to be cleaned thoroughly to remove harmful chemical residue, insecticides, pesticides, or simply just handling contaminants. Organic fruits and vegetables are preferred to lessen the chance of having these residual impurities.

Organic means grown in natural environments free of harmful chemicals.

Organically grown fruits and vegetables will provide the best natural taste and nutrition, while store bought is perfectly acceptable as well.

Smoothie or Juice

Is it a smoothie or is it juice? Here is the difference:

A smoothie has the pulp of the fruits and vegetables mixed in with the juice. Juice does not have the pulp, only the juice.

The smoothie and juice both contain the same nutrient quality, but do not contain the same consistency. The pulp from juicing can be used for a variety of different things to include compost for your garden, dehydrating to make chips, making pet food or treats, freezing for a cool snack in the summertime heat, making soup broth, or whatever your clever mind can conjure up.

Why Do You Want To Juice Fast

To begin your juicing phase, ask yourself why you want to start. Do you want to lose weight? Give your body more nutritional support? Cleanse your body from many years of junk food damage? Realize how close you can be with your spiritual side and fast for personal and private reasons? Whatever your answer to the question *"why"*, it is yours and personal. There is a good chance that it will be a more successful course if you realize why you want to begin a fast of any sort. There is no need to convince yourself that you want to do this – you only need to understand the reason why. This will help with setting your goal of how long you want to fast.

Set Starting Goals

Begin by setting a goal of how long you want to juice fast. Do you want to do a short course of three to five days to get a feel for it? Do you want to have a longer goal of thirty, sixty, or more days? Again, I cannot stress enough how important it is to get the approval of your physician, especially if you are going to attempt a longer juice fast. When I tried my first juice fast, I did three days just to see how it would make me feel and if I could break the habit of hand-to-mouth eating. I was able to do this with little to no side effects. There are some detoxifying side effects that you will experience, but these will gradually go away and you will be back to your normal self in no time. I have provided a section on this as well that you can use for reference. Documenting your journey from beginning to end will help you understand what your likes and dislikes were, motivations that worked or did not work, and more importantly, what the outcome was. Did you reach your goal? What kept you motivated? What fruits and vegetables did you use? How long did you juice fast?

Preparing Your Mind, Body, And Soul

Well, I think you deserve a pat on the back for making it this far – congratulations. The toughest part is yet to come. Most of you have families at home, young children, spouses, teenagers, parents who may still live with you, or extended family or friends residing in your home that will not be taking part in your decision to do a juice fast. These members of your household will still need to eat during the day and someone will have to prepare their meals for them. Grilling their steaks, frying their chicken, baking their birthday cakes, making their apple pies, and even if you are not the person who has to provide the meals for the members of your family; you will still be able to see and smell these ongoing palate teasers. I was lucky enough to have my husband agree to take his part in the juice fast in the evening, at dinnertime. This made it easy for me to stay on track and not have to cook so many meals or be tempted to break my fast early. There were times when it would have been easier to fry chicken and gobble it up than to juice kale and cucumbers to drink, but reflecting back on my goals I had set for myself kept me on track. Wanting to mentally break the junk food trap my body had been forced to fall into and lose weight in the process was the trigger I needed to keep me from harming my body any more than I already had.

There will also be friends and family who will not understand why you are taking part in a juice fast. They will have questions and will look to you for answers. Educate yourself well enough to be able to answer these questions. This is a great time to share your aspirations and goals with those who are asking and maybe they will join you on your path to getting healthy!

How Will You Motivate Yourself

Motivation is the key to a successful juice fast. Inspire yourself to stay on task and keep an eye on your goals that you have written down and read them over and over. If necessary, watch *"Fat, Sick, and Nearly Dead"* over and over a couple times or keep it on hand to watch when you need the extra support during the rough times. The mental concept of not bringing food to your mouth to eat is one of the hardest things I had to overcome. Once I mastered this, I was on my way to changing my life around and my nutritional habits. I found that using a straw aided in this to begin with, as well as alternating between warm, room temperature, and even some cold juices. Being able to answer other potential juicers inquisitions is also a great way to motivate yourself and them. If you know the answer to the question before it is asked, you have done your homework! Keep a journal from day one until you end your juice fast. Make note of when you feel like throwing in the towel, times of the day that you are at your strongest or weakest to continue on your juice fast, what triggers you to succeed, what triggers you to fail; all of your notes will aid you in your continued lifelong healthy habits. Also, keep track of the good triggers with the *"bad"*, as these will help motivate you on your future juice fasts. If you write it in your journal, it will give you a tool to use for yourself and to share with others as well. Find a friend to juice fast with; this will give you some extra support and someone to talk to as well.

Exercise And The Juice Fast

When I first started my juice fast, I was told the necessity for exercise is paramount for a successful juice fast. In the beginning phase, during the first two to three days when your mind and body are struggling with the changes, it is best not to take on too much physical exercise right away, but to begin exercising slowly. Keep your exercise progress in your journal as well. What exercise did you do and for how long? I began with taking short walks several times a day and yoga, and then progressed to exercise that was more physical when my body was better able to handle it. Walking, swimming, stair climbing, steps, crunches, all of these exercises are great for your body and help keep your energy level up as well. *As with exercise of any sort, please make sure to get the approval of your physician prior to beginning a new or physically demanding regimen.* Your body may not be able to handle very much to begin with, but you can always build up to a better more physical exercise regimen as you progress.

Keep A Journal Of Your Progress

You have heard me mention repeatedly to keep a journal of your juice fast, all notes including good and bad need to be documented here. This can be something as simple as a three-ring binder, stenographer's tablet, composition book; whatever you want to use to keep track of your juice fast progress is perfectly acceptable. Here are some of the items you will want to keep track of:

Your beginning, middle, and ending body measurements, daily recipes (including what you like and dislike), your exercise (including what type of exercise and for how long), notes about your emotional health and wellbeing, detoxification symptoms you are experiencing, how you are feeling that day, start and end dates, and any other journal notes you want to enter for that day.

Keeping track of this information in your journal will give you a very valuable tool to use in the future when you want to juice fast again. This will also be a great tool to share with others who are still skeptical about starting their own juice fast and have come to you for words of encouragement or looking to you for education and experience. I have included a sample to help get you started.

Before Juicing

This section will give you step-by-step instructions on how to juice and will provide you with the information necessary to get you heading in the right direction.

Gather together all of the supplies you will need to begin juicing. I start my morning with my juicer (remember this can be any type of juicer you want, whatever fits your finances and needs or is best for you. No single specific juicer is required, just what you prefer). I also have a fruit and vegetable strainer that I use to keep the bigger particles out of my juice, a glass pitcher, a Mason jar for whatever juice I have remaining, a spoon to stir with, a knife to cut with, a small garbage bag, another small container to keep my pulp in, and a 16-ounce glass.

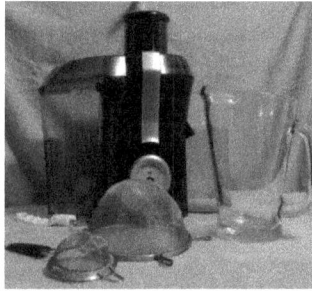

Next on the list comes the vegetables I am going to start my morning with – yep I start my day with veggies, not fruit. The preferred ratio of fruits and vegetables is 80 percent more vegetables than fruit for each beverage. So, I use lots of veggies and only a little fruit.

I clean all of my fruits and vegetables and have them ready to run through the juicer. Some are sliced, skinned, or cored, while others go in the juicer whole. This will vary on your flavor preference. Usually citrus fruits will have a very bitter flavor if you juice them with their skins on.

I also keep ginger root, parsley, cayenne pepper, and garlic on hand as well for flavoring. Use spices in moderation just like you would for regular cooking, as you do not want to over-power your juices.

Once everything is ready, I can begin my juicing for the morning. The preparation can be done at your own discretion, but I did all of mine at the time I juiced. Again, this is your preference and is not required to be any specific way – do what fits you best!

I have my recipes on hand and build my juice, making sure that I will have about 16 to 32 ounces of juice for breakfast, lunch, and dinner. I prepared my juice for each meal of the day prior to drinking it. I wanted my juice fresh and this prevented wasting fruits and vegetables.

Take Your Body Measurements To Compare

Prior to beginning your juice fast – measure your body. Start at the top and work your way down. I included my measurements at the beginning to give you a reference point of how my numbers decreased and these are part of my journal. You will want to measure:

Bust line circumference (or nipple line), waistline (I called it my belly button waistline as that was my focal point), hips, each leg, and maybe even each arm as well. Also, document your beginning weight.

I included the dates for each set of measurements in my journal as well, again another piece of information you will want to look back on.

Preparing The Fruits And Vegetables For Juicing

When you begin juicing, you will want to select nutritious fruits and vegetables to get the best value out of every drop you drink, both financially and for your health. Select fruits and vegetables that you like and also a few that you dislike.

Mix what you dislike in with what you like to take advantage of the nutritional benefit while disguising them. Adding zucchini or yellow squash in with your juice disguises well. Neither can be tasted and they provide tons of nutrients and lots of juice too.

Getting your daily supply of vitamins will be so easy with juicing that you will wonder how you ever managed before!

Washing

When you purchase your fruits and vegetables, they will need to be washed properly to remove all of the harmful chemicals that are on them. There is a cleaning solution of vinegar and water (*use equal parts of vinegar and water*) that you spray onto your fruits and vegetables, let the solution stay on for about 15 to 20 minutes, and rinse off in cool water. Do not use hot water to clean your vegetables as this may shrivel the skins and start the withering process early. You can also *mix 2 cups water, 2 tablespoons of baking soda, 2 cups vinegar, and the juice from a whole lemon into a spray bottle. Spray on fruits and vegetables, let sit for approximately 10 to 15 minutes and rinse with cold water.* Whichever solution you choose, remember to wash your hands and the surface you will be preparing your juices on as well.

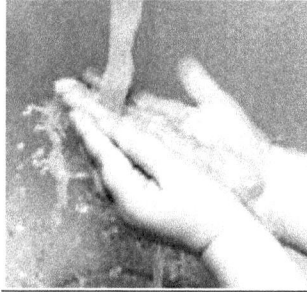

Storing The Juice

Fresh juice needs to be stored in an airtight glass jar, like a Mason canning jar. Fill the jar completely to the top and cover tightly. The fresh juice can be stored in the refrigerator for up to 48 hours, but should not be stored any longer or it will lose its nutrient value. You can freeze fresh juice for up to 72 hours if you need to, but the thawing process will take away some of the nutrients. The best advice I can give is to consume the juice you make for the day to get the most benefit from it and only store your juice in the refrigerator if you absolutely have to. Making what you need and using it right away will help keep all of the nutrients fresh and there is less waste of the fruits and vegetables.

How To Juice

Select your supplies, set your goals, get motivated, prepare your journal, get your measurements, and get ready to juice. The more motivated and educated you are about your juice fast, the easier it will be to stay on track and know what to expect. You will need to drink approximately 16 to 32 ounces of fresh juice a day (if you are eating one meal per day) to roughly 64 to 72 ounces maximum (if you are not eating one meal per day and only consuming juice) of fresh juice per day, so be sure you purchase enough supplies to last the length of your juicing goal. You will also need to remember that your body will be going through a variety of stages when it begins to start cleansing your cells, as we mentioned earlier. These can range from unnoticeable to very noticeable, depending on how your body reacts to the juice fast. Drink lots of water as well. Water helps keep your system hydrated, so make sure you are drinking enough water to maintain your body. The estimated amount of water you will need to drink will depend on you. The average amount is 2 to 3 liters per person, but this will fluctuate depending on the weather, amount of exercise you do, and your environment. Drink enough fluid to help keep you adequately hydrated and if you are thirsty, grab another sip or two. I made it a goal to try to drink as much water as juice. If I drank 64 ounces of juice, then I *tried* to get in 64 ounces of water as well.

During Juicing

During the juicing phase, your body will be going through some changes. These changes will be noticeable and may have the ability to affect your medical issues. You may experience a runny nose, headache, fever, or even sore throat. There are medical studies taking place every day to suggest that a plant-based diet will help with some types of medical ailments. When you are educating yourself on the juicing process, please pay special attention to any medical condition that you have and research how juicing will influence your ability to come off some medications, lose weight, and feel better overall. Getting the proper nutrition and staying away from junk food will help to keep you healthier; it sure cannot hurt you by any means. This is coming straight from a 40 plus year junk food-aholic too!

While you are juicing you will notice that your taste for junk food will diminish over time. After watching "*Fat, Sick, and Nearly Dead*", you will wonder why you ever ate all those greasy cheeseburgers and fries, and like me will probably never touch another one.

While we are all humans and tend to be imperfect, we will at times "fall off the wagon", but do not worry – just pick yourself up, dust off your knees, and get back to eating healthy fruits and vegetables again.

Symptoms Of Detoxifying Your Body

While you are cleansing your body's cells during your juice fast, you will experience some symptoms that can be minimal to major. The first one to three days are usually the worst and this is when hunger is the most intense. During this time, you may experience symptoms of dizziness, headaches, slight nausea, foul breath, glazed or glassy eyes, a coated tongue, lightheadedness, and possibly even diarrhea. Preparing yourself will help minimize the symptoms. Gradually break yourself away from the bad habits of eating junk food and eating more fruits and vegetables *prior* to beginning a juice fast and your body will be able to tolerate the changes easier than hitting it full force. Approximately one week to ten days prior to beginning your juice fast, try to limit your intake of caffeine, sugars, dairy, tobacco products, and alcohol. This will help keep the symptoms minimal.

Day three to seven are a bit easier to handle. This is when your body begins to adjust and the symptoms of your body getting healthier by the day will change. You will notice your hair being softer, your skin looking better, and your whole body feeling better – from the inside out. It will be very evident how much your body appreciates you feeding it nutritious fruits and vegetables compared to filling it with junk food. You may notice little spots on your skin where the toxins inside your body are wanting out and these will take on the appearance of small pimples or eruptions. During this time, your body will begin to produce more white blood cells and begin to rest its digestive tract. You may feel pain in different areas of your body as the toxins are being expelled. If the pain becomes severe, you may need to seek the advice of your physician. During the release of the harmful toxins, your body will take on the appearance of the common cold; your nose may run, you may cough, you may run a slight fever. These are all common symptoms and the best advice I can give you is to push through them; they will not last long. I experienced these symptoms during my juice fast and was able to continue juicing without having to stop my progress. You may have a different outlook and may need to stop your juice fast if the symptoms become too much to handle.

Remember to document what you are experiencing for future reference, especially in the event that you need to stop your juice fast earlier than expected.

Day eight to two weeks, this is when your energy picks up and you will begin to feel better. The varying symptoms will fade or even resolve completely by this phase. The only downside will be old injuries may begin to bother you again. When you were originally injured, your diet was not as it is now and the human body is very resilient, so with you eating healthier and living a better life; the old injury is still trying to heal properly and this is where the pain will come from. Not everyone experiences the same symptoms, so do not let this deter you from juicing longer than three days.

Day fifteen up to day 30 is when the juice fast plays the most significant role in cleansing your cells.

At this phase, your body will be adjusted to the juicing process and your body will be healing from the inside out. This is the phase that we all try to reach and where we get the most benefit While not everyone is able to juice for a full 30 days, the shorter fasting phases will have a healthy impact on your body as well. So no need to worry if you are not able to go for a full 30 days. Document your juice fast from beginning to end so you can see where you need to change things around to have a better juice fast on the next go-around.

These symptoms will all vary depending on you and your body. Not everyone will experience the same ill effects, but the potential is there for you to have the above-mentioned signs and you should be prepared for any or all of them.

Should You Stop Prior To Completing Your Goal

There is no shame or harm in stopping your juice fast earlier than you anticipated. There are many people who will find that they will need to stop for medical reasons, financial reasons, or whatever reason they have. This does not mean you failed at your juice fast; this simply means you stopped earlier than you had set your goal to achieve. This is where documenting your progress will play a significant role in helping you pick up and begin again. You will know the basics of how to begin, what to do, and how to do it.

Juice fasting does not have rules to follow or numbers to count, so never feel pressured to stop. There is no harm in this. Just pick up where you left off. Eating properly will become a life-long desire that you will want to partake in.

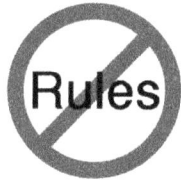

After Juicing

After you complete your juicing goal that you set for yourself, you will see how beneficial the fast was for your mind, body, and soul. You will look better and feel better, but you will also realize how your eating habits have been affected as well. Most generally, those who begin a juice fast will change their eating habits for the better and remain eating healthy diets. There is no harm in eating foods that are not 100 percent plant-based. The harm comes when you eat foods that are not *good for your body*. Eating meat and dairy products is normal and expected; after all, we are humans, but eating in moderation and understanding how the food you eat affects your *whole* body will help you to establish better eating habits for you and your family. Eating more fruits and vegetables will provide you with the nutritional support to maintain a happy healthy lifestyle and keep your cells cleansed in the process.

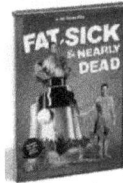

How To Stop The Right Way

When you have completed your goal and it is now time for you to stop your juice fast, this has to be done with as much thought as starting. It is important to remember that your body has been free from solid forms of food while you have been nourishing it with fruit and vegetable juice. When you re-enter the solid foods back into your diet, do so in small amounts and start with softer foods such as mashed potatoes or steamed vegetables so your body can adjust back to digesting solid foods again. Even if you have set a goal of a three-day juice fast, please re-introduce solid foods slowly back into your meals. If you consume solid foods too quickly when stopping your juice fast, this can be harmful if not fatal to those who have medical ailments prior to beginning the juice fast such as diabetes or heart-related issues. Set all of your juice fast goals from beginning to end – how you start is as important as how you stop.

Common Symptoms Of Stopping The Juice Fast

Stopping your juice fast will surely cause your body to react to the changes. The most common symptoms of stopping a juice fast are stomach pains and diarrhea. Re-introducing solid foods back into your diet will make your body adjust accordingly so please remember to take this phase slowly as well. You may also experience the opposite and have constipation, which can be helped by drinking more water. Watch for dehydration symptoms, if you have either diarrhea or constipation treat these accordingly. If you are having difficulty with either, to the extent that no matter what you do to try to resolve them is not working, please seek medical attention.

Now that you have completed your juice fast, try to remember why you started to begin with. Try to refrain from eating fried foods, dairy products, red meats, and other foods that are not healthy for you unless it is in moderation. Never gorge yourself and overeat foods that are not healthy for your body. Try to stick with healthy options and drink lots of water.

How Long To Fast

How long to fast will be one of the first steps in setting your juice fast goals. You will need to prepare yourself for the length of time you will be juicing and the amount of time required to stop the juice fast. The length of time generally is a matter of personal preference and can be three, five, ten, fourteen, thirty, sixty, or ninety days. Eating one small meal along with your juice fast will also play a role in the length of time you fast. If you are not eating and only nourishing with juice, will also be another determining factor. When you have your consultation with your physician, this would be a good time to set the length of your juice fast and begin your process of preparing, documenting, motivation, and beginning.

Setting Exiting Goals

It is important to set exiting goals too. What will your goal be when you are finished fasting? Will you reward yourself with a new outfit? Will you share your juice fast strategy with others? Will you change the way you eat and what you eat? My exiting goal was to keep the weight I had lost off, which was easy to do since I did not go back to eating junk food as I had been eating prior to beginning my juice fast. My diet now consists of 80 percent plant-based nutrition and I am not willing to change back to the "*old*" way again. I have inspired others to begin a juice fast and they too have changed their eating habits and have been able to keep their weight off and help others accomplish this same goal. Setting an exit goal or goals is important so you know what you have to look forward too when you are done fasting. This too should be part of your journal and part of your preparation start juicing. As they say – everything has a beginning and an ending, so plan everything out from beginning to end.

Motivating Others To Juice Fast

Beginning a juice fast is a personal goal to begin with. You will want to achieve your own goals and share your accomplishments with others. Having a friend share with you in your fasting journey is a great concept and one that everyone should have. My husband did a partial fast with me and never discouraged me in any way to do my juice fasts. He encouraged me every day to stay on track and keep focused on what my goals were – my very own juicing coach and motivator! There are others who will not accept your thoughts, goals, or concepts of juicing – no matter how hard you try to convince them that it is perfectly healthy. Having the hand-to-mouth repetition of eating is what they are used to and what they prefer. While on the other hand, there will be those who will latch onto your thoughts and travel along this journey with you, which is a great feeling! Keep in mind that juicing is not for everyone, but for those of us who understand it and want to participate, there are others out there that have the same motivation. Doing your research and educating yourself will provide you with the information you will need to locate other juicers and point you in the right direction of sharing your thoughts and ideas. One of the biggest things that juicers share is recipes. I have documented a variety of recipes that I use personally and will share them here with you. Some I have tried and some I have gathered through research. Work with others to create juice recipes that you too can share with others.

Maintaining Your Weight After Juice Fasting

Once you have completed your juice fast and before you begin another, here are some ways to keep the weight loss you have achieved during your juice fast:

- Drink plenty of water to stay hydrated.
- Eat a good, healthy breakfast
- Use portion control
- Prepare your own meals
- Resist cravings
- Avoid alcohol and smoking
- Get proper rest
- Quit starving yourself
- Exercise

The exercise you do daily can be a great way to keep the weight you have come to like now that you are done fasting. Walk before meals for approximately 10 to 15 minutes to get your body activated and walk again after you eat to boost your metabolism. You should exercise a minimum of 30 minutes every day. You can scatter your 30 minutes throughout the day, but get in a minimum of 30 minutes. Doing more than 30 is better, but it is a good place to start. Once you get acclimated to 30 minutes daily, raise up to 45 minutes, and eventually up to 60 minutes. Mix up your exercise and have fun with it. Document your achievements in your journal to see how you have progressed and where you need to work harder.

Keep an eye on how much you are eating as well. Use portion control to help guide you through the day. Keep your meat intake to approximately the size of the palm of your hand, eat more fruits and vegetables, starchy and carb filled foods need to be about the size of your fist; no bigger. Think of a smiley face when it comes to proportioning food on your plate. The meat/starch/carb portions would be ¼ the top portion of your plate and the fruits and vegetables would fill in the remainder or about 50 percent of your plate.

Prepare your own meals. When you eat at a restaurant, the proportions they give you are tremendous and not healthy. You can eat half of your meal and take the other half home with you. When you cook your own meals, you know what they were cooked with as well. You can decide which oil to use, how much flavoring is needed, and control the amount you eat a lot easier too. If you do go out to eat, ask for your salad dressing on the side; dip your fork in it and then take a bite of salad. Also, do not fill up on the bread and dinner rolls waiting for your meal to arrive.

Get enough rest. If you get hungry take a quick nap instead…this helps keep your binge eating to a minimum. Cortisol kicks in when you are stressed and produces more belly fat, so keep an eye on your stress level. A few good ways to reduce stress can be meditation, yoga, walking, praying, talking to others, relaxing your muscles, working in your garden, or reading a book. Try to get six to eight full hours of sleep per night. While this may be difficult for some, it can be helpful to document your progress.

Cravings – we all have them and we all get them. You can help lessen your urge to binge eat and cravings by drinking water or distracting yourself. Pay attention to what triggers the craving and keep track in your journal. The same methods used to lessen your stress can be used to distract yourself from whatever you are craving. Are you craving what you see on television commercials? Do you get hungry at two in the afternoon and crave sugar to help keep you awake?

Another way you can keep track of your diet is to wait until you are hungry to eat. When your belly growls or you get the hunger pangs, and then is the time to comply with your body. Your internal dinner bell will let you know when your body is seeking your attention. The key is to eat slowly and savor your food, bite for bite. Stop eating before you are too full. You want just enough to satisfy your hunger. Use portion control and do not overindulging on your favorites. Sit down to eat and do not eat in front of the television or while you are on the computer.

These are bad habits that will lead to overindulging and swaying from your strategy to maintain your goal weight loss. Always eat breakfast. When you skip breakfast your body has not had a chance to wake up inside and this will cause you to feel more tired and sluggish as the day progresses. Pay attention to your body and listen to what it tells you.

Purchase healthy foods to eat. Do not stock up on junk food and tell yourself that you will not sway and give into eating all of the brownies or chips. Your eyes will see these snacks, your nose will smell them, and then your mind tries to convince your body that it needs them. Ugh – nothing like throwing all of the time and energy you spent cleansing yourself from the inside out *away* for a few minutes of sugary temptation. Why would you want to go backwards and not forward now that you have made it this far? Keep an eye on what comes in your house and kick the bad foods out. Read the labels on the items you purchase and educate yourself.

MEASURE EQUIVALENTS				
Cup =	Fluid OZ =	TBSP =	TSP =	Milliliter
1C	8 oz	16 Tbsp	48 tsp	237 ml
3/4C	6 oz	12 Tbsp	36 tsp	177 ml
2/3C	5 oz	11 Tbsp	32 tsp	158 ml
1/2C	4 oz	8 Tbsp	24 tsp	118 ml
1/3C	3 oz	5 Tbsp	16 tsp	79 ml
1/4C	2 oz	4 Tbsp	12 tsp	59 ml
1/8C	1 oz	2 Tbsp	6 tsp	30 ml
1/16C	.5 oz	1 Tbsp	3 tsp	15 ml

Summary

In summary, juicing is a great way to cleanse your body from all of the harmful foods you have consumed for many years. This is not a weight loss program that has you counting carbs or going to meetings, but one that allows you to stay healthy and feel great in the process. The weight loss alone may be one of the main reasons you want to begin a juice fast or maybe just refresh your system internally. Cleaning your digestive tract of harmful ingested foodstuffs you have added into it for so long is truly the most gratifying feeling. Being able to lose weight, have better-looking skin and hair, staying healthy enough to possibly decrease the amount of medicine you take daily, getting the proper nutritional support from your diet, and boosting your energy are all great reasons for a juice fast.

There is no set way to juice; it all depends on you and what you are hoping to gain in the end. There is no rulebook to follow and no one to answer to when you prepare yourself for your juice fast. By documenting all of your goals and information from start to finish, you will have a very valuable tool to use when you are prepared to begin juicing again and to share with others.

Researching and educating yourself with information will provide you with the knowledge you will need to start your juice fast. Learning what fruits and vegetables taste well when the juice is blended together, which recipes are the healthiest for you, making your own recipes, sharing recipes with other juicers, learning where to find others who share this common interest with you, and eventually those who will want to learn from your example. The learning never ends. Take the time to find the answers you are looking for, you will be greatly rewarded the results of what you have learned.

Some Questions I Have Been Asked

Here are some of the questions I was asked during my juice fast...

- Do you like the juices you make? Yes, but some are better than others. I was sure to write down the recipes I enjoyed so I could use them again.
- Are all of the juices green and taste like fresh cut grass? No, the color depends on what fruits and vegetables you mix. The flavor is a mixture of the different fruits and vegetables you combine. If it need mellowed out a bit, put an apple it in to smooth out the taste. You can also add spices like ginger or garlic to add flavor too.
- Does it take a lot of fruits and vegetables for a juice fast? This depends on how long you are going to fast. I generally shop for supplies once a week to keep my foods fresh and so I do not run out.
- How expensive was your juicer? I spent fifty dollars for it online at Amazon.com. I could have found a cheaper one, but I liked this one due to the large opening where the fruits and vegetables are inserted. It is also very easy to clean and reassemble. It has safety features too and will not run if everything is not properly placed.
- Do you have to pay so much for a juicer? No, go with whatever works for you. There are juicers you can literally spend thousands of dollars on and juicers you can buy at a dollar store. You will find one that matches your needs and finances, and that is the one you will more than likely purchase.
- Can you only juice organic fruits and vegetables? No, any fruits and vegetables will work. The organic fruits and vegetables provide more nutritional benefit. They are not a requirement for juicing. They also are grown without harmful chemicals added to them, so are healthier for you as well.
- Do you only have to drink juice or can you eat food too? You can juice for two of the three meals a day and have a small meal mixed in. This is the beauty of a juice fast; you

can do whatever works best for you. When I started, I drank juice only for the first few fasts I did, then I ate one meal a day to my regimen.

- Can you keep doing a juice fast while you travel? Yes, we travel quite a bit in our motorhome and I still juice when we go. You will find that this actually helps when you are juicing to give you a variety of fruits of vegetables too. What is locally grown at your home may not be the produce grown elsewhere, so it helps mix it up a bit.

- Was your doctor ok with you juicing? Every one of my physicians I spoke to about juicing encouraged me to go ahead and do whatever worked for me; they were completely fine with this and supported my efforts 100 percent. They did tell me to pay attention to my body and if I had any problems to let them know.

- What were some of your symptoms you had when you were juicing? I experienced a little nausea the first couple of days, some diarrhea, one day of being lightheaded, and glassy eyes, but I only had this for two days and then by day three I was feeling great! You may not experience the same symptoms I did and may have something completely different. Only you know your body and can tell when something just does not fit right and when something does.

- What recipes do you like best? I like recipes that are not typical that are born from mixing things together that you would not expect and still have a great outcome. The greener the veggie; the better it is for you. The sweeter fruit juices may cause you to gain weight so be careful how much of this you drink. I try to stay away from adding to much fruit to my vegetable drinks and only add enough to make them taste good. Adding a little bit of fruit will change the flavor of your drink very nicely. Adding spices helps too.

- If you had one secret you could share about juicing what would it be? To remember to rinse your mouth out and frequently. The mouth is a good place to hide offensive smells and bacteria. When you think of it, swish some water around in your mouth to help keep hydrated and lessen the worry of offensive breath.

- Did you ever feel like stopping earlier than you wanted? Yes, right before vacation, but I knew that everything I had accomplished up to that point would have been a waste of time and effort, so I pushed through and motivated myself to reach my goals. Juicing is definitely not for everyone and requires willpower on some days to get through the "*rough spots*". Be tough and push through – you can do it.
- How do you keep from grabbing a little bite of food when cooking for others? I had a juice on hand to drink or sip on *while* I was cooking and every time I was provoked to want a bite, I took a sip of my juice instead. I also kept snack fruits and veggies on hand in case the cravings would get intense.
- How do you get others to understand and not think you are being foolish for wanting to start juicing? You cannot make others accept juicing; they do this through understanding what it is and making their own mind up from there. Being open-minded and staying educated helps when others start asking questions. Just be prepared to give them honest answers and share some of your goals with them. They are only curious because they do not know what it is, usually. Once they understand and are well informed, they most generally will accept it.
- I have type 2 diabetes; will doing a juice fast help me to get rid of some medicines I take for this? Juice fasting has been shown to help some medical conditions such as diabetes. It has even been known to reverse it in some people. While not all medical conditions are alike, just like people, each condition is different. My advice would be to talk to you physician about this.
- What type of medical ailments will juicing help? Juicing can help with a variety of medical conditions such as migraine headaches, some forms of arthritis, diabetes, constipation, anemia, obesity, skin conditions, gallstones, asthma, and diarrhea. While I am not a physician and not able to say that all of these conditions will be cured with juice fasting; I can tell you that it is best for you to talk with your doctor about this. They have the knowledge and expertise to point you in the right direction.

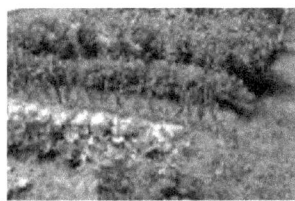

Recipes

Minty Strawberry and Pineapple
1/2 large pineapple, peeled and cored
1-1/2 cups strawberries
2 pears
30 mint leaves

Mixed Berry Mint
2 cups blueberries
2 kiwi
2 cups strawberries
2 cups packed mint leaves

Blackberry and Mint
1/2 large pineapple, peeled and cored
2 cups blackberries
2 kiwi
2 pears
30 mint leaves

Pineapple Orange Juice
2 oranges, including rind, cut in half
1/2 ripe pineapple, peeled and cored
3 carrots
1/2 lemon, peeled

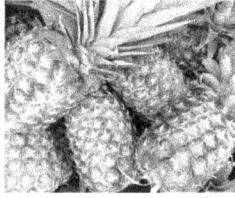

Beet-Orange Juice
2 oranges
3 red beets
1 apple

ABC Juice
1 apple
2 beets
3 large carrots
1/2 inch piece of ginger, peeled
1 handful of spinach or kale

Purple Juice
6 cups grapes
1 apple
1 inch piece of ginger, peeled
1 cup blackberries

Apple-Melon Juice
2 apples
1 cantaloupe, peeled and deseeded
1 honeydew, peeled and deseeded
2 handful of kale or Swiss chard leaves

Green Fruit Drink
2 cups packed beet greens
2 handfuls Swiss chard, kale, spinach
1 apple
1 pear
2 cups strawberries

Sunset Evening Juice
1 large sweet potato
1 carrot
1 red bell pepper
2 beets
2 apples
1 orange
1 pear

Green Orange Juice
2 cups romaine hearts
2 apples
1 orange
2 celery stalks
1 cucumber

Green Carrot Juice
1 green apple
3 handfuls spinach
3 handfuls kale leaves
4 large carrots
1 inch piece of ginger, peeled

Carrot-Lemon-Lime Juice
1 lemon, peeled
1 lime, peeled
2 pears
2 apples
2 carrots
1 inch piece of ginger, peeled
2 cups cabbage

Green Pineapple Juice
1 large pineapple, peeled and cored
2 handfuls kale
1 handful spinach
1 cucumber
4 celery stalks
1 inch piece of ginger, peeled

Apple-Cabbage-Carrot Juice
2 apples
1/4 cabbage
2 carrots
1 inch piece of ginger, peeled
1 handful Swiss chard leaves
1/2 lemon, peeled

Greeny Green Juice
2 handfuls kale
2 handfuls spinach
1/2 cucumber
4 celery stalks
2 apples
1 inch piece of ginger, peeled

Citrus Tart Juice
3 cups cranberries
2 -1 inch pieces of ginger, peeled
3 oranges
2 grapefruits
2 limes

Green Ade Juice
1 green apple
3 handfuls spinach
2 handfuls kale
1/2 cucumber
4 celery stalks
1/2 lemon, peeled

Green Tart Juice
2 handfuls kale
2 handfuls spinach
1 cucumber
4 celery stalks
2 apples
1 inch piece of ginger, peeled
1/2 lemon, peeled

Beet Mint
2 beet
2 carrots
1 apple, cored
1/4 cup mint

Green Plum Juice
4 plum tomatoes
1 large cucumber
2 celery stalks
1 red bell pepper
1/2 small onion
2 cups packed parsley leaves and stems
1 lime

Tomato Tart
4 tomatoes,
5 celery stalks,
3 carrots
1 inch piece of ginger, peeled
1/2 lemon, peeled

Almost Everything Green Juice
1 handful romaine hearts
1 handful collard greens
1 handful spinach
2 handfuls parsley
1 handful kale
2 to 3 celery stalks
1 inch piece of ginger, peeled
1/2 lemon, unpeeled
Pineapple Ade
1 large pineapple, peeled and cored
1 cup seedless grapes
1/2 inch piece of ginger, peeled
1 apple

Vitamin Ade
1 bunch parsley
1 handful kale
1 handful spinach
1 inch piece of ginger, peeled
1 small bunch of lettuce
1 apple or 2 carrots (optional)
6 broccoli florets

Mango Berry
1 mango
1 cup strawberries
1 apple
1 pear

V31 Juice
3 beets
3 carrots
3 celery stalks
4 plum tomatoes
4 cups packed parsley leaves and stems
1 jalapeño pepper, ribs and seeds removed
12 red radishes
1 inch pieces of ginger, peeled

Watermelon Juice
4 cups watermelon
1 inch piece of ginger, peeled
1/4 cup mint

Berry Ade
1 cup raspberries
1 cup strawberries
2 oranges
1/2 pineapple

Orange Sips
2 carrots
1 apple
1 pear
1/2 lemon, peeled

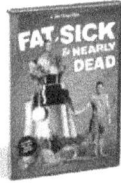

Journal Entry Sample

In this section, you will want to include your beginning, middle, and end measurements. You may also want to add a few extra sets of measurements in there as well, depending on how long you will be fasting. You will want to include your goal measurements as well. You will want to document what motivates you to begin the juice fast, what exercise you will do, what juice you had, how you felt, and how you are motivated. All of this information can be used to reflect back on when you want to juice again. Document your experience from day one through until your exit off your juice fast and watch how much you will change your body and self to being a healthier you!

Final Goal Measurements

(This is what you want your measurements to be when you are done with your juice fast)

Length of time: ___ days

Bust line: ___ inches,
Belly button waistline: ___ inches,
Hips: ___ inches,
Left leg girth: ___ inches,
Right leg girth: ___ inches.
Weight: ___ pounds.
My Body Measurements for Day One

(These are your current day one body measurements)

Date __/__/__

Bust line: ___ inches,
Belly button waistline: ___ inches,
Hips: ___ inches,
Left leg girth: ___ inches,
Right leg girth: ___ inches.
Weight: ___ pounds.

Day One Information

I am beginning my juice fast on __/__/__ for approximately ___ days. Dr. _____ has agreed that this is acceptable and I am medically able to begin.

I am motivated to start juicing for the following reasons:

_____
_____
_____
_____

_____

_____

The juice I will start with:

_____

_____

_____

_____

_____

The exercise I will do today:

_____

_____

_____

_____

_____

I experienced these symptoms while juice fasting:

_____

_____

_____

_____

_____

Notes:

Fruits

This is a partial list of some of the common fruits used in making juice recipes and what vitamins they contain (this information was gathered from researching online through popular medical websites) …

Acaí – Contains vitamin A, B, C, E
Apple – Contains vitamins A, B, C, E, K
Apricot – Contains vitamins A, C, K
Avocado - Contains vitamin A, B, C, E, K
Banana - Contains vitamin A, B, C, E, K
Blackberries - Contains vitamin A, B, C, E, K
Blueberry - Contains vitamin A, B, C, E, K
Cantaloupe - Contains vitamin A, B, C, E, K
Cherries – Contain vitamin A, B, C, E, K
Clementine – Contain vitamin A, C
Coconut – Contain vitamin B, C, E, K
Cranberry - Contains vitamin A, B, C, E, K
Currant - Contains vitamin A, B, C, E
Date - Contains vitamin A, B, C, E, K
Dragonfruit   Contain vitamin A, B, C, E
Eggplant – Contains vitamin B, C, K
Elderberry – Contains vitamin A, B, C
Fig – Contains vitamin A, B, C, K
Gooseberry - Contains vitamin A, B, C, E
Grapes - Contains vitamin A, B, C, E, K
Grapefruit - Contains vitamin A, B, C, E
Honeydew - Contains vitamin A, B, C, K
Kiwi - Contains vitamin A, B, C, E, K
Kumquat - Contains vitamin A, C, E
Legume - Contains vitamin A, B, C, K
Lemon - Contains vitamin A, B, C, E
Lime - Contains vitamin A, B, C, E, K
Loganberry - Contains vitamin A, B, C, E, K
Mandarin - Contains vitamin A, B, C
Mango - Contains vitamin A, B, C, E, K
Mulberry - Contains vitamin A, B, C, E, K
Nectarine - Contains vitamin A, B, C, E, K
Oranges - Contains vitamin A, B, C, E

Papaya - Contains vitamin A, B, C, E, K
Passionfruit - Contains vitamin A, B, C, E, K
Peaches - Contains vitamin A, B, C, E, K
Pears - Contains vitamin A, B, C, E, K
Pineapple - Contains vitamin A, B, C, E, K
Plum - Contains vitamin A, B, C, E, K
Pomegranate - Contains vitamin B, C, E, K
Prunes - Contains vitamin A, B, C, E, K
Raisin - Contains vitamin B, C, E, K
Raspberries - Contains vitamin A, B, C, E, K
Starfruit - Contains vitamin A, B, C, E
Strawberries - Contains vitamin A, B, C, E, K
Tangerine - Contains vitamin A, B, C
Tomato - Contains vitamin A, B, C, E, K
Watermelon - Contains vitamin A, B, C, E, K

Vegetables

This is a partial list of some of the common vegetables used in making juice recipes and what vitamins they contain (this information was gathered from researching online through popular medical websites) ...

Acorn squash - Contains vitamin A, B, C
Artichoke - Contains vitamin A, B, C, E, K
Arugula - Contains vitamin A, C, K
Asparagus - Contains vitamin A, B, C, E, K
Bamboo shoot - Contains vitamin B
Bean sprouts - Contains vitamin B, C
Beet - Contains vitamin A, B, C
Beet greens - Contains vitamin A, B, C
Beetroot - Contains vitamin A, B, C, E, K
Bell pepper - Contains vitamin A, B, C, E, K
Black beans - Contains vitamin A, B
Black-eyed peas - Contains vitamin A, B, E, K
Bok choy - Contains vitamin A, B, C, E, K
Broccoli - Contains vitamin A, B, C, E, K
Brussels sprout - Contains vitamin A, B, C, E, K
Cabbage - Contains vitamin A, B, C, E, K
Carrot - Contains vitamin A, B, C, E, K
Cauliflower - Contains vitamin A, B, C, E, K
Cayenne - Contains vitamin A, C
Celery - Contains vitamin A, B, C, E, K
Chickpeas - Contains vitamin A, B, C, E, K
Chili pepper - Contains vitamin A, B, C, E
Collard greens - Contains vitamin A, B, C, E, K
Corn - Contains vitamin A, B, C, E, K
Cucumber - Contains vitamin A, B, C, E, K
Eggplant - Contains vitamin A, B, C, E, K
Endive - Contains vitamin A, B, C, E, K
Garlic - Contains vitamin B, C, E, K
Ginger - Contains vitamin A, B, C
Green bean - Contains vitamin A, B, C
Kale - Contains vitamin A, B, C, K, E
Kidney beans - Contains vitamin B, C, E, K
Leek - Contains vitamin A, B, C, E, K

Legumes - Contains vitamin A, B, C, K
Lettuce - Contains vitamin A, B, C, E, K
Lima bean - Contains vitamin B, E, K
Mushrooms - Contains vitamin B, C, D
Mustard greens - Contains vitamin A, B, C, E, K
Okra - Contains vitamin A, B, C, E, K
Onion - Contains vitamin A, B, C, E, K
Parsley - Contains vitamin A, C, K
Parsnip - Contains vitamin B, C, E, K
Pea - Contains vitamin A, B, C, E, K
Pinto beans - Contains vitamin B, C, E, K
Potato - Contains vitamin A, B, C, E, K
Pumpkin - Contains vitamin A, B, C, E, K
Radish - Contains vitamin A, B, C, K
Rhubarb - Contains vitamin A, B, C, E, K
Soy beans - Contains vitamin B, C
Spinach - Contains vitamin A, B, C, E, K
Squash - Contains vitamin A, B, C, E, K
Sweet potato - Contains vitamin A, B, C, E, K
Swiss chard - Contains vitamin A, B, C, E, K
Tomato - Contains vitamin A, B, C, E, K
Turnip - Contains vitamin B, C, E, K
Yam - Contains vitamin B, C, E, K
Zucchini - Contains vitamin A, B, C, E, K

How To Educate Yourself

When it comes to learning, do what works best for you and helps you retain knowledge. I use the internet to research various topics and make notes for the information that I want to keep. While you are researching online, enter keywords (words used to describe what you are looking for) into your search engine to get more information such as:

- Juice fasting

- Juice recipes

- Medical benefits of juicing

- Social networks of juice fasting

- "*Fat, Sick, and Nearly Dead*" documentary

- Jointhereboot.com

- Weight loss with juice fasting

- Where can I order organic fruits and vegetables

- Where can I buy a juicer

- Healthy exercises

- Learning yoga

Learn as much as you can about eating healthy and staying in shape. Read books. There are multiple books available on Amazon and in your local library. Go to agricultural meetings in your community to find out more about growing organic gardens and where to find them in your neighborhood. This will provide lifelong healthy habits for you and your family. Inspire others to be as healthy as they can be too. Join networks of people who have experienced juicing, those who strive to be healthy, and those who can help you along your way to being healthier.

CHALLENGE

My challenge to each of you is to find someone to do a juice fast with or try it on your own. Begin with a short three, five, or seven day trial first and see how far you can go. Start by documenting your measurements and see how much weight you can really lose. You will see the inches decrease along with your weight. All while cleansing your cells and body in a very healthy and nutritious way, without counting numbers or attending meetings. If this is your first time juice fasting, you may not see a dramatic change in your weight with only a three-day course, so give it the extra two days and see if you notice a change then. Be honest with yourself and with your juice fast by setting goals and keeping good records of your journey. See how many recipes you can share with the network of friends you have made while doing your research.

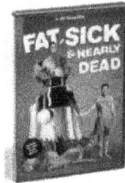

On A More Personal Note

I want to thank you for taking the time to read all of the wonderful information I have prepared for you here. Whether or not you begin a juice fast, I am pleased to know that you have taken the time to educate yourself on a great option for losing weight and cleansing your body from the inside out.

A diet or change in your daily lifestyle takes courage and commitment, as well as full understanding of the change you are planning to make. I congratulate you on making the decision to take the challenge and make yourself healthier.

I encourage you to continue educating yourself and learning as much as you can about the food you eat, how your body uses it, and what you can do to make a change in the way you eat.

From me to you…"*thank you*"!

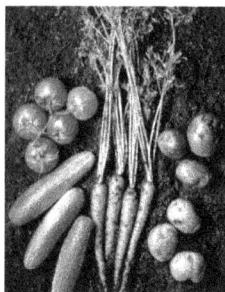

Sites Of Reference

The following are some websites I use for research and referencing material –

- WebMD - http://www.webmd.com/

- Mayo Clinic - http://www.mayoclinic.com/

- Healthline - http://www.healthline.com/

- Livestrong - http://www.livestrong.com/

- Join the Reboot - http://www.jointhereboot.com

- PubMed - http://www.ncbi.nlm.nih.gov/pubmed/

- Google - http://www.google.com/

- CDC - http://www.cdc.gov/

- Medline Plus - http://www.nlm.nih.gov/medlineplus/encyclopedia.html

- Vitamins - http://www.nlm.nih.gov/medlineplus/encyclopedia.html

I also strongly encourage you to see the documentary *"Fat, Sick, and Nearly Dead"* by Joe Cross. He shares his own personal amazing story and juicing knowledge with you. You can get more information about this documentary by going to http://www.jointhereboot.com or typing "Join The Reboot" into your search engine.

Special permission has been received to use the name of Joe Cross and his documentary "Fat, Sick, and Nearly Dead" in this book.

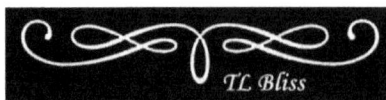

ABOUT THE AUTHOR

"I started writing poems when I was just a little girl. I never did much with anything I wrote other than read it a few times and then put it away. Over the years, everything I had written was lost or destroyed, but the memories I had still lingered on in my mind. We all struggle with things deep within us and outside of us that intrigues our senses enough to want to tell the world about it; why not share what stimulates us and sparks our emotions through a book."

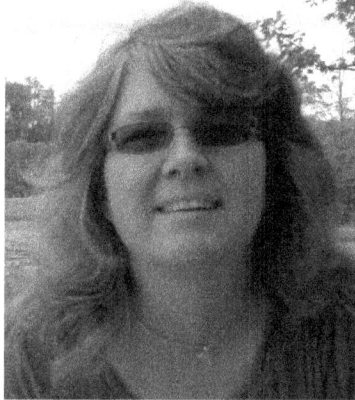

Visit www.tlbliss.com for more information and links to purchase other stories written by TL Bliss.

www.ingramcontent.com/pod-product-compliance
Lightning Source LLC
Chambersburg PA
CBHW070811210326
41520CB00011B/1905